DEDICATION

I dedicate this book to my two lovely daughters. May you both always have the courage and strength to overcome whatever problems that you may encounter as you take your journey call life.

Table of Contents

Publishers Notes 2

Dedication 3

Table of Contents 4

Chapter 1- What is Anxiety and Stress? 5

Chapter 2- Anxiety by Definition 12

Chapter 3- Possible Causes of Depression and Anxiety 16

Chapter 4- Don't Be a Victim of Anxiety 19

Chapter 5- How to Go About It 31

Chapter 6- Alternative Way of Treating Anxiety 39

Chapter 7- Don't Let Anxiety Attacks Dictate You 45

About The Author 48

CHAPTER 1- WHAT IS ANXIETY AND STRESS?

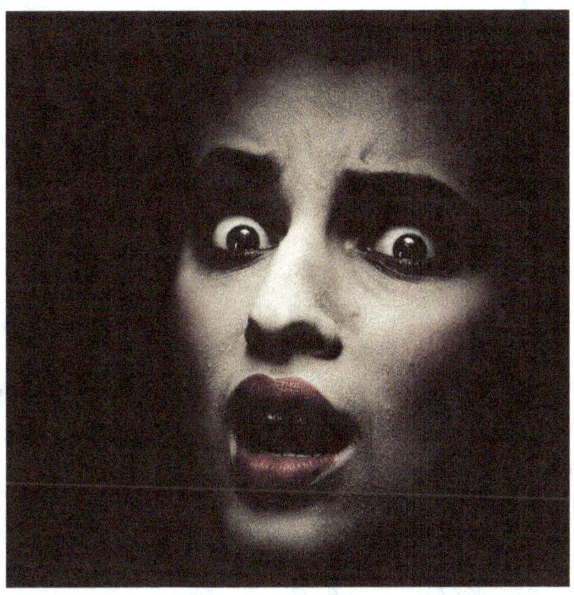

Unless you have been lost at sea over the past ten years, you have probably not only heard about depression and anxiety, but also heard about them on a daily basis. You have also most likely watched countless advertisements about this that appears to be a "new disease." Depression and anxiety are nothing new. They have been good buddies that have followed some folks around since the beginning of time. It is just now we are free to talk about it.

Why are we free to talk about it now when psychiatry has been around for nearly 150 years? Probably because there is a lot of money to be made in treating these illnesses with pharmaceuticals. And pharmaceutical companies want to sell drugs that are supposed to cure depression and anxiety so that they can make money.

What are depression and anxiety? Are they diseases or just weaknesses to which certain individuals fall prey? Those who are proponents of modern psychology feel that they are diseases that must be treated with medication and therapy. Those who are against modern psychology feel that this is a state of mind that can be overcome with strong will. Who is right? This book will teach you not only about depression and anxiety and the different levels of this disorder, but also a bit about the history of depression, the different ways that they manifest themselves, how to tell if you need treatment and many different ways to treat both disorders.

Most information that you read about depression or anxiety is created to sell you a certain cure or idea regarding these matters. Very few are objective when it comes to their reporting. Most will be slanted one way or another. If you read information from a pharmaceutical company, for example, they will tout the different medicines that are available for depression and anxiety.

Then there are the all natural cures that will tell you how dangerous medication is. Then there is this book. This is you all comprehensive book about depression and anxiety. Here you will learn everything there is to know about depression and anxiety in easy to understand language. You will also visit with some people who have suffered with depression and anxiety and see how they helped themselves. By learning all of the facts about depression and anxiety, you will be better prepared to make a decision regarding your own treatment or the treatment of a loved one.

Depression

Everyone gets the blues all of the time. No one is happy, happy, joy; joy all of the time unless they are on drugs. If you are like most people, you have had days where you have felt depressed. You may feel a little weepy or feel sorry for yourself. This can be related to an incident that has happened in your life or for no particular reason. Some say that we get depressed because of the weather.

There is even a mental disorder called "Seasonal Affective Disorder" that is supposed to be triggered by lack of light.

Depression is tough to define. It can be different things for different people. A person with a negative personality, for example, may seem depressing a lot more than a person who is always positive. This is why it throws you for a loop when the person who is always positive jumps off a bridge and the person who is always negative are still around. Depression is not always easy to spot and is different for each individual.

Clinical Depression is a serious illness. People who are clinically, severely depressed usually try to commit suicide at one point in their lives sometimes they succeed. They find it difficult to maintain jobs or relationships. They tend to look at the glass half empty, which is an old cliché but rings true with those who suffer from depression.

People who are severely depressed for long period of time are diagnosed with clinical depression. This is one of the major reasons why many people are disabled in the United States. Back pain and clinical depression claim most of the disability claims in the US each year.

A person who is clinically depressed cannot "snap out of it." It can be frustrating for loved ones to watch a person in this condition as the natural instinct is to shake them and tell them to "snap out of it." We tell them how grateful they should be for everything that they have and point to people who have it far worse. We may as well be talking to a wall. The clinically depressed person cannot just decide to not be depressed one day. They realize that there are others far worse off than them, but it doesn't make them feel any better.

This type of "therapy" that is often given to the depressed can do more harm than good. It makes the person who is suffering from depression feel as though he or she is being self indulgent.

Some people take it a step farther and accuse the depressed person of "seeking attention." This is also damaging to the psyche of a depressed person, particularly because depression is so closely related to self esteem issues.

Depression comes in many different forms for each individual. It will most likely manifest itself by making a person who suffers from this illness lethargic and not interested in doing every day things. The person who suffers from depression may not like to do anything. They may sleep too much or not at all. They may feel angry and lash out at people a lot of the time. They may also feel angry with themselves.

In some cases, a person will go through the motions of their everyday life without any joy. They seem almost like an empty shell. They look for any type of relief from this state that they can get, which is one reason why so many people abuse drugs and alcohol.

You may or may not realize that someone is suffering from depression.

A person may appear listless and not have any energy or they may put on a really good front. Two sad cases of people who had depression are Marilyn and Jimmy.

Everyone used to call Marilyn "The Grim Reaper." She was always dark and moody. She used to talk about death a lot of the time and also drank to excess. She went from doctor to doctor to try to get help for her depression.

Marilyn used to say that depression was like a dark cloud that followed her around. If you knew Marilyn, you could almost see the cloud. She walked slumped over and never seemed happy. Even after she began seeing the doctor for severe depression, she still never seemed to spruce up.

Marilyn's family said that she had been depressed most of her life.

Coincidentally, Marilyn's mother had committed suicide when Marilyn was a little girl. Apparently, her mother was also clinically and severely depressed.

When she was 30 years old, Marilyn took an overdose of barbiturates that had been prescribed for anxiety and washed them down with whiskey. A friend found her body the next day after phone calls went unanswered. None of her friends or family was that shocked that Marilyn killed herself. She didn't even leave a note.

Jimmy was one of the most popular kids in high school. He was a gifted athlete who had a full scholarship to his dream college. He had a ton of friends in school and a girl who he also liked. All his life, things seemed to come easy to Jimmy.

He exceeded at sports which made him well liked throughout his school career. It also made his parents very proud of him.

Jimmy's parents had just gotten divorced after a long and strained marriage. Jimmy and his sister were both upset about the divorce and missed their father who had moved out of the family house. But Jimmy appeared happy on his last day of school, the day before high school graduation.

Looking back on that day, most of his friends realized that they had been left clues. They just didn't pick up on them. That day, when Jimmy went home, he parked his car in the garage and left it running while shutting the garage door. His sister was at a friend's house.

Jimmy knew she was going to be gone and that his mother was at work. He knew no one would find him until it was too late and he was right.

Jimmy left a note. It told his parents that he had been depressed for some time and that his suicide had nothing to do with the divorce. He felt that he had had a good life and, at the age of 17, felt that it was time for him to "move on."

The news of the suicide devastated Jimmy's family as well as his friends. The entire school was affected. Thousands of people went to the wake where his stunned parents sat in disbelief. His sister, who found his body, was also there. The entire family was in shock as was the school. No one saw it coming.

The sad thing was that Jimmy's school as counselors. They have classes and seminars about depression. They have teachers that are taught how to look for "the signs." The kids have access to counseling whenever they want it. Jimmy was the fifth student to kill himself in the last four years at the school.

Depression is not always evident. There are people who walk around like Marilyn all of the time but have no intention of ever killing themselves. There are people who appear to have everything going for them and then suddenly do something drastic, like Jimmy. You can never tell.

Only the person who is experiencing depression can help themselves.

Parents of a person who is depressed can take them to the doctor and the doctor may even prescribe medication, but if the young person will not take the medication, or, when they reach a certain age, refuse to take the pills, they cannot be helped. They may even, like Jimmy, realize that there is a lot of attention placed on depression and decide to hide it so that no one finds out.

Contrary to what you may think, not everyone who suffers from depression has suicidal thoughts. Most just have thoughts of emptiness and despair. They don't want to die but don't' want to live, either. They may try to get help for themselves, like Marilyn, or may deny that there is anything wrong at all with them, like Jimmy. In short, depression has many different forms and takes on a different meaning for each person.

No one is sure why some people suffer from chronic depression and others do not. Most of us, however, at one time in our lives, will deal with depression of some sort.

How you deal with depression is up to you. Hopefully, the more you realize that it is an illness that can be treated by a number of different ways, you will try to fight the depression and not give in to the dark feelings that may overpower you.

CHAPTER 2- ANXIETY BY DEFINITION

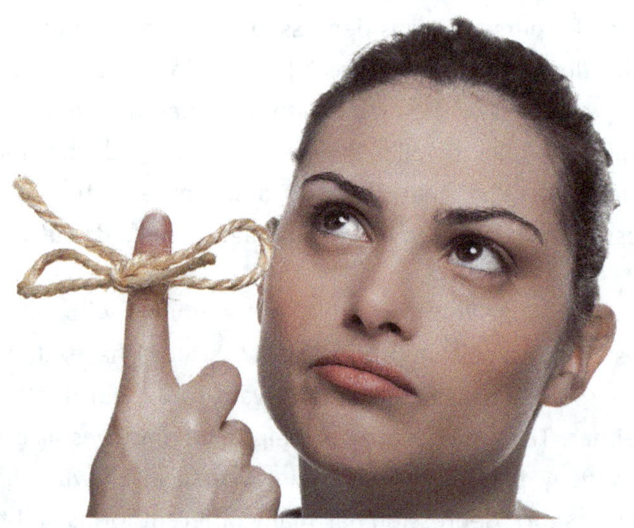

Whereas depression tends to make someone lethargic and not feeling like they want to do anything, anxiety makes them jumpy, nervous and in a state of fear. Anxiety is fear of the unknown. It is easy to put a name on this disorder. Anxiety disorder manifests itself in a variety of different ways. The root of anxiety, most psychiatrists believe, is depression. People who are depressed often also experience anxiety. These two diseases go together like peanut butter and jelly.

Some of the ways that anxiety manifests itself include obsessive compulsive disorder, anorexia nervosa, social anxiety disorder, phobias, general anxiety disorder and others. These are all different syndromes that also manifest themselves in different ways. And they all have one thing in common - it is all about control.

People who are depressed often suffer from anxiety and vice versa. Excessive worrying is one way that obsessive compulsive disorder manifests itself. Usually a person with obsessive compulsive disorder worries about germs or the house burns down or the doors being unlocked. He or she performs rituals to give them a bit of control over this worry. The worry is usually not about the doors being unlocked or the house burning down but a fear of the unknown. People who experience this illness tend to have more problems with obsessions and compulsions during chaotic times in their life when everything is out of control.

Anxiety often triggers panic attacks, or anxiety attacks. This can make someone feel as though they are having a heart attack. They feel all of the symptoms of a heart attack and usually end up in the emergency room of the hospital. When they find that they have had an anxiety attack, they are relieved.

Anxiety attacks can be really dangerous. Some people actually faint during such attacks from hyperventilating. This can happen anywhere, even when driving. Others may ignore true heart attack symptoms thinking that they are having an anxiety attack. Anxiety also raises the blood pressure of most individuals. It makes a person feel as though they are crawling out of their skin.

Anorexia nervosa is actually a condition that stems from low self esteem and depression and can be considered an anxiety disorder. A person with this condition has the delusion that they are fat, even though they are rail thin. They continue to starve themselves. Singer Karen Carpenter suffered from this disease that eventually ended up killing her. After the starvation, the body can no longer take the strain and the heart gives out.

Anorexia is all about control, as are other eating disorders. A person suffering from this disorder usually feels things spinning out of control and looks for something she can control. Most of the people who suffer from anorexia are young women, college or high school aged. They usually start out a little overweight and someone makes a remark about it. This does not do much for their self esteem which is usually already fragile because they also suffer from depression. They diet a little because of the hurtful remark and lose some weight. Viola!

Most psychiatrists will say that anorexia is a separate disorder, but it has roots in anxiety and depression as well. Anxiety and depression can usually be found in anyone with a mental disorder. They are pretty much the parents of all mental health issues, but different issues are more serious than others and the anxiety and depression manifest themselves differently.

According to Dr. John Bolton of Palos Park, Illinois, depression and anxiety usually are the result of low self esteem. A person who suffers from these disorders sees themselves as worthless. The feeling of low self esteem makes them feel powerless and causes depression. The constant need for some sort of controls over their environment and feeling of being powerless to help those causes the anxiety.

They are afraid most of the time and cling to a certain fear in order to feel "safe." The fear, or phobia, is usually something that is imagined in their head and in many cases, does not even exist.

Sigmund Freud, who is considered the father of modern Psychiatry, felt that depression was the result of stifled creativity. Freud noted that many depressed individuals were also highly creative. There are those who agree with Freud's theory and those who take issue.

Today, the feeling is that people who suffer from depression have a chemical imbalance in their brains that can be "cured" with artificial serotonin that is given in pill dosage. People who have anxiety are usually treated with tranquilizers by the medical community as well as therapy. Most doctors today subscribe to the theory that people with depression and anxiety have a physical illness that is due to a chemical imbalance in their brain. They also believe there may be a genetic link. Others disagree with this theory and believe it is the result of low self esteem or problems in childhood. Still others blame society and poverty for people feeling depressed.

In short, medical science has a lot of theories about why so many people suffer from anxiety and depression, but no clear cut answers. But there is one thing that you will rarely hear a doctor say, and that is "I don't know."

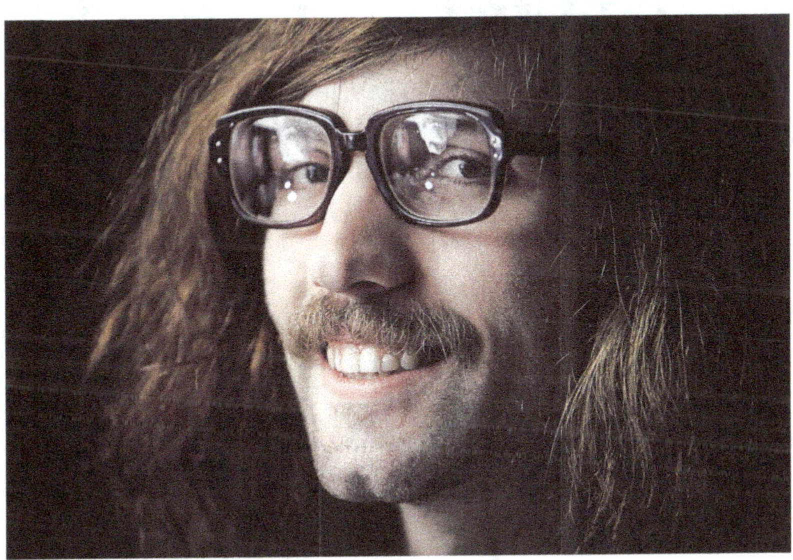

Chapter 3- Possible Causes of Depression and Anxiety

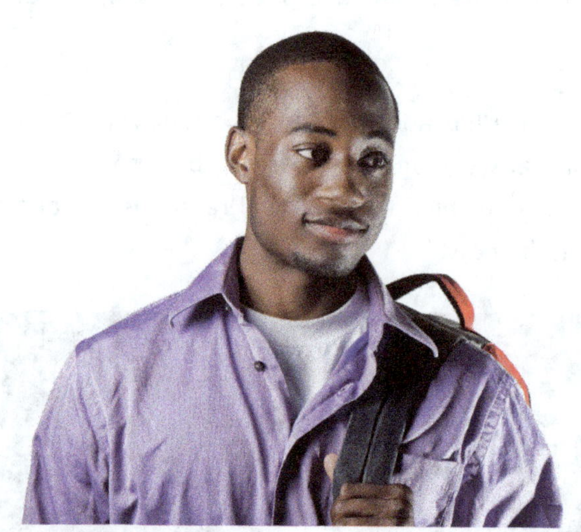

As mentioned in the last chapter, there are disputes in the medical field regarding the causes of depression and anxiety. Some psychiatrists are very Freudian in their belief that this is all about stifled creativity. Others blame genetic makeup. When we talked about Marilyn, we noted that her mother also committed suicide. It appears that mental illness, such as depression and anxiety, can be inherited.

Other doctors blame society. Poverty will cause depression. Take a look at people who are living in poverty for most of their lives. Their faces reflect blankness as if they don't care about anything. You can see it from their behavior. The drug use is rampant in poverty stricken areas, as is alcohol use. Why do people think this occurs? It is because the people who are so despondent, who are subjected to misery on a daily basis, tend to look for a quick fix and begin to self medicate. Our answer, as a society, is to arrest them for using drugs.

Some doctors actually blame drugs and alcohol for the depression and anxiety. They are few and far between, while alcohol does nothing to help those with depression and are, in itself, a depressant, it is the symptom of the disease of depression, not the cause. Alcoholics, like most addicts, suffer from low self esteem, depression and are looking for some way to control part of their environment.

Then there are those in the psychiatric field who believe the illness is physical. We have a chemical imbalance of serotonin in our brains that must be alleviated by taking medication, called SSRIs. This discovery coincides with the discovery of SSRI medication and promotion by the pharmaceutical companies. There are no medical tests that can determine if those with depression suffer from a chemical imbalance in the brain. As it stands now, this is just another theory as to why some people are prone to depression.

If you ask a priest or a religious person, they will tell you that depression and anxiety are due to a lack of faith. People who have faith in a particular religion seem to suffer less from depression and anxiety. But is the religion the reason why they do not suffer or is it their form of self medication? Just like some people get addicted to alcohol and drugs and use them as a crutch to get through life, others use religion. This is a much less dangerous crutch to an individual, unless they become fanatical to the point where they are causing harm to others.

Some people believe we all have a degree of depression and anxiety. That anxiety is the fear of the unknown that exists in all of us. The thing we fear is death - the one thing that no one wants to face but we all must sooner or later. It can also trigger depression. Freud also said we had a death wish and a life wish. Perhaps depression is a signal of our death wish.

There are many different theories on why people become depressed and anxious. The theories will also dictate the cures or treatments. A medical doctor, for example, will be quick to prescribe drugs. A Freudian psychiatrist may be more apt to try a cognitive therapy. Therapists, hypnotists, acupuncturists, herbalists, priests, doctors and the guy at the car dealership all have different theories on depression and all have an idea of how it should be treated. Most people in the United States, however, go to the doctor when they are feeling depressed.

Chapter 4- Don't Be a Victim of Anxiety

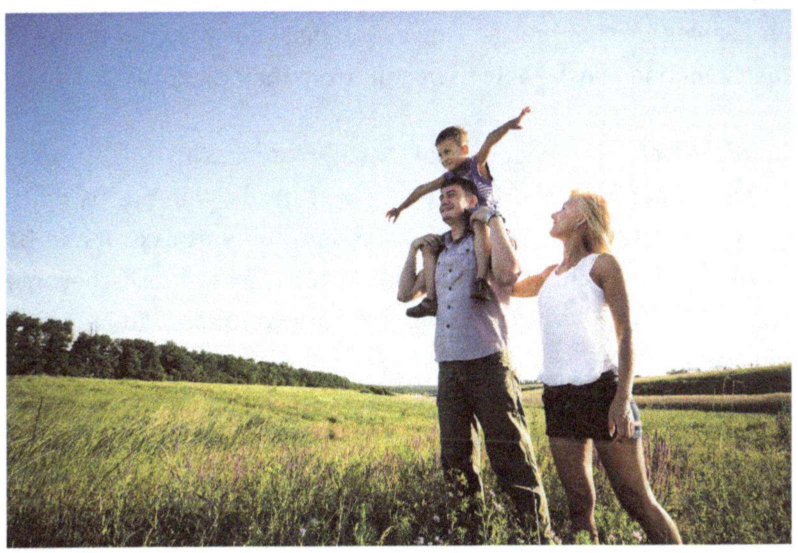

There is no certain group on this earth that is a target for anxiety and related attacks or disorders. So, with that said, who do you think suffers from this? Well, it could be anyone. It could be in your family, your friends, co-workers or anyone that you may know.

A lot of times, it could be those that you know and you would have never thought in a million years that they would suffer from something like this.

Unfortunately, these attacks are usually kept secret and not disclosed. This is one of those "sweep under the rug" embarrassment moments. This is not something that is talked about out in the open. Some people will acknowledge dealing with this when they are caught in the act and can't fake it.

Believe it or not, there are people such as politicians and even Hollywood celebrities who suffer from anxiety attacks and related conditions. However, they pay their publicists and others to keep it out of the public eye.

They don't want to be in the spotlight because they have to work on keeping up their image. However, what they may not realize is that someone may be able to benefit from their disclosure.

Unfortunately, for people that have to deal with this, anxiety attacks affect and tend to interfere with those who are trying to live a normal life. If you have excessive anxiety attacks, it can be related to a psychiatric condition. When these attacks become serious and they last a long time, they are considered to be out of the norm.

With the symptoms of an anxiety attack, the brain relays messages to other parts of a person's body. Certain parts of the body, such as the lungs and heart work overtime while the anxiety attack is happening. The brain ends up releasing a lot of adrenaline.

Different Forms/Kinds of Anxiety that You need to Aware of

Generalized Anxiety Disorder (GAD)

Generalized anxiety disorder, or GAD, deals with people that are constant worriers and are always tense. The thing about this is that there really isn't a cause for this, nor is anyone or anything at fault to provoke it. They look for the worst and are always extremely worried about work, family health and money. They even feel anxiety in the course of their normal day.

If this pattern is consistent for at least six months, a person can be considered as suffering from GAD. They feel that they cannot stop worrying even though the concern is not as great as they make it out to be.

It's difficult for them to relax, they are easily startled by people or noises and they have a hard time focusing. Sometimes they cannot sleep at night or wake up in the morning on their own. Here are some other symptoms that contribute to generalized anxiety disorder:

• Feeling tired

• Aching muscles

• Irritable

• Nauseated

• Sweaty

• Lightheaded

• Shortness of breath

• Frequent trips to the bathroom

• Shaking or trembling

• Hot flashes

If they don't have a high anxiety level and still suffer from generalized anxiety disorder, they can still be employed and be able to interact socially with others. However, if they have GAD on a higher scale, they may have trouble doing and completing simple tasks that others would take for granted.

Close to seven million American adults suffer from generalized anxiety disorders. There are more women (about twice as many) than men that are dealing with this. Even with that, the risk reaches its peak starting at childhood and going through the middle age years. Studies have shown that there are some genes that contribute to people getting GAD.

There are other anxiety disorders that happen in conjunction with GAD, such as substance abuse and depression. If treated properly, the person affected can overcome their worries with whatever problems they are dealing with.

Social Anxiety Disorder

Social anxiety disorder, which is also known as social phobia, happens when a person is extremely self-conscious and anxious. It happens every day in different social situations. They are extremely fearful of being watched.

They are also fearful of being judged by others. They try to be extremely careful and go out of their way to not do things that could cause them embarrassment.

For a while, they are extremely fearful prior to a situation that they feel can become a disaster. It can become so bad that they lose focus and can't think straight. With social anxiety disorder, they can allow this fear to cause them to lose focus.

It doesn't matter whether it happens at school, work or at home. Having social anxiety disorder can make it difficult for the person affected to cultivate relationships with others.

With social anxiety disorder, it may be somewhat difficult for people to get over their excessive fears and concerns. This is true even if they know that what they feel is not realistic. Some will try to make amends.

Even then there is a feeling of anxiety and they don't feel comfortable when they are around other people. Then they are overly concerned of how others thought of them after the encounter.

A person could be in a social setting (for example, at dinner with someone or more than one person) and they will experience anxiety because they are fearful. They will sweat a lot, blush, shake, or find it difficult to hold a conversation with other people at the table. They always seem to feel that other people are watching them.

There are over 15 million adults in the United States alone that suffer from social anxiety disorder or social phobia. For the most part, this condition begins as a child and can continue through adolescence.

There are some studies that say genetics plays a part in this. This condition is often coupled with depression or other anxiety disorders or attacks. It is not a good idea for those affected to treat themselves with medication. It could make the situation worse. This is better treated with professionals that are experienced in this field.

Obsessive Compulsive Disorder

People that deal with obsessive-compulsive disorder, or OCD, constantly have thoughts that can make them upset. In order to get their anxiety under control, they use compulsions (rituals). However, the tables end up turning on them because the rituals take control over their mind.

For instance, there are some people that are obsessed with being clean. They are known as "clean freaks". Of course, it's a good practice to want everything to stay clean, but they can get to the point of being overly controlling about germs or dirty surfaces.

They have a compulsion to wash their hands continuously. They don't want any germs or dirt to touch their hands. When they go to the bathroom, they will take a paper towel to open and close the door, just to keep from getting germs on their hands.

If people that have OCD don't feel like they look their best, they will look in the mirror several times until they feel they are presentable. They don't want to feel as though they look out of place among others.

These actions provide them with a temporary release of the anxiety that they have been feeling. People with this disorder are always compelled to check things repeatedly, or make sure that things are in the same place repeatedly.

Sometimes, they are obsessed with ideas of violence or harm to others. They also have thoughts of crazy things that people would not normally think about. There are times when they feel they have to hoard and keep things that they don't need.

There are some that have rituals in their home. One of the more common ones is checking the stove several times before they leave to make sure it is off. Having obsessive-compulsive disorder can turn into havoc and an unwelcome interruption when it happens on a daily basis.

When a person is engrained with obsessive-compulsive disorder, they know what they are doing doesn't make much sense, but they don't look at their behavior as something that is abnormal.

There are over two million adults in the United States that have obsessive-compulsive disorder. This condition does not stand out on its own. It can be combined with things such as anxiety disorders or attacks, depression or eating disorders.

This disorder affects women and men almost equally. It usually starts as a child or it can start in the teen years or even as an adults. Through research, there is an indication that OCD can happen through genetics. At least of third of all adults in the United States start out with OCD as a child.

The symptoms of obsessive-compulsive disorder can come and go at any time. If it really gets bad, it can severely affect a person from acting in a normal capacity and doing certain tasks. It's a good idea for those that are dealing with this not to use alcohol or drugs to calm them down. It just makes the situation worse for them.

There are certain treatments and medications that can be used to ward off obsessive-compulsive disorder. They can help people that are in fear or anxiety to be desensitized to what is going on around them.

Post-Traumatic Stress Disorder

Post-Traumatic Stress Disorder or PTSD happens when someone has suffered something that included harm of the body or implied the threat of harm. The person who gets PTSD may have been harmed, or it may have been someone close to them.

PTSD is commonly known in regard to veterans who served in a war. However, there are other things, such as a rape, kidnapping, abuse, vehicular accidents, plane crashes or natural disasters such as hurricanes or floods.

Those that suffer from Post-Traumatic Stress Disorder can be easily startled. They also have no feeling for those who they used to have a close relationship with. They start to have less interest in things they used to do. They show less affection, are increasingly aggressive and show more of the irritable side.

They try to block out things that remind them of that traumatic event instead of working through it. If the event was something that someone else deliberately acted on against them, then PTSD will greatly affect them.

Nightmares can haunt them and they start to see flashbacks such as sounds, feelings and images of what happened. There are sounds that can remind them of that event. For instance, if a door slams, then that could mean that someone has you trapped in a room and ready to pounce on you with their abuse.

It could by physical or verbal. Some people don't realize that verbal abuse is just as bad, if not worse than physical abuse.

Keep in mind that everyone who has been traumatized will not experienced PTSD. Some people are able to cope with what happened and move on. There are others that need therapy and medication to deal with their issues.

PTSD can start a few months after the event or incident. It could last for a few more months, or continue through the years. In order to be officially classified as PTSD, the symptoms have to continue for at least a month. There are some who end up having PTSD as a chronic condition.

There are over seven million adults in the United States that are dealing with Post-Traumatic Stress Disorder. It can start from the childhood years and work its way up to adulthood. There are more women that suffer from this than men. PTSD is also combined with substance abuse, depression or other anxiety disorders or attacks.

Panic Disorder And Panic Attacks

Panic disorder is considered to be an illness. Symptoms include feeling suddenly terrorized, feeling faint, and pain in the chest or feeling smothered. Panic attacks fall under the panic disorder condition and are prone to some of these same symptoms, plus others. When someone is having a panic attack, there are thoughts that are unrealistic or they fear that they are no longer in control or a situation.

With panic disorder, a person can also experience depression, or substance abuse. If these conditions are attached to their panic disorder, they should not be treated together. Sometimes they will feel sad or won't want to eat. They may not be able to sleep or only sleep for a few hours. They don't have much energy to do anything and they cannot maintain focus.

Panic Attack

A panic attack is when a person has a fear or apprehension that is sudden or intense. There is usually nothing wrong and no one is in danger. Panic attacks can happen suddenly, last for a few minutes, and then it's over. There are others that last longer than a few minutes or there may be more than one and they follow behind one another.

There are three types of panic attacks:

• Spontaneous –these panic attacks occur with no warning. There is nothing that could possibly bring it on. Even if a person is sleeping, they can still experience a panic attack.

• Situationally bound – these panic attacks happen when there is a situation to which a person has been or will be exposed to. They are considering triggering or provoking the panic attack. For instance, if a person hears a car backfire, it could remind them of when they were in the military and fighting a war with ammunition.

• Situationally predisposed – these panic attacks can happen when there is a delayed reaction. The attack doesn't always occur right away. There are some instances where people may immediately have an attack, and other instances it is delayed or it may not happen at all.

Panic attacks are defined as having at least four or more symptoms:

• A choking feeling

• Lightheaded or dizzy

• Shaking

• Trembling

• Shortness of breath

• Accelerated heartbeat

• Pain in chest

• Numbness

•Chills

•Feeling of going crazy

•Nauseated

•Sweating

•Feelings of detachment

If a person experiences less than four symptoms, they can still be classified as having a panic attack, but it would be called a "limited symptom" panic attack. A person can have a panic attack at any time. It can even happen when they are sleeping. It has affected millions of adults in the United States.

However, there are more women that experience panic attacks. In fact, women experience panic attacks twice as much as men do. Panic attacks can start in the late teen or early adult years.

There are people that have frequent panic attacks and allow themselves to become almost helpless. There are some places where they will have stay away from because it can trigger another attack.

Or a person may not be able to participate in some activities, like going shopping and related outings. Most of the time, they are confined to where they live and won't go out unless someone else is with them.

This condition is called agoraphobia, which is when a person is fearful of open spaces or being out and about by themselves. If they seek help early for this, the progressive treatment can be successful.

It is a very treatable anxiety disorder and will respond to most medications or therapies that are provided to them. Medication and/or therapy can help the affected person to alter the way that they think in order to rid themselves of fear and anxiety.

If you have frequent panic attacks, you may have a panic disorder. Panic attacks become a panic disorder when the condition becomes chronic. You life can be in serious danger, along with others.

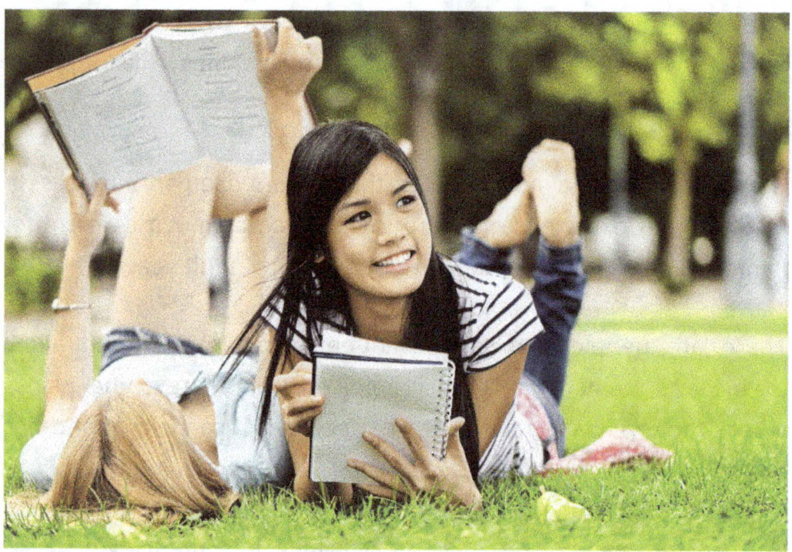

Chapter 5- How to Go About It

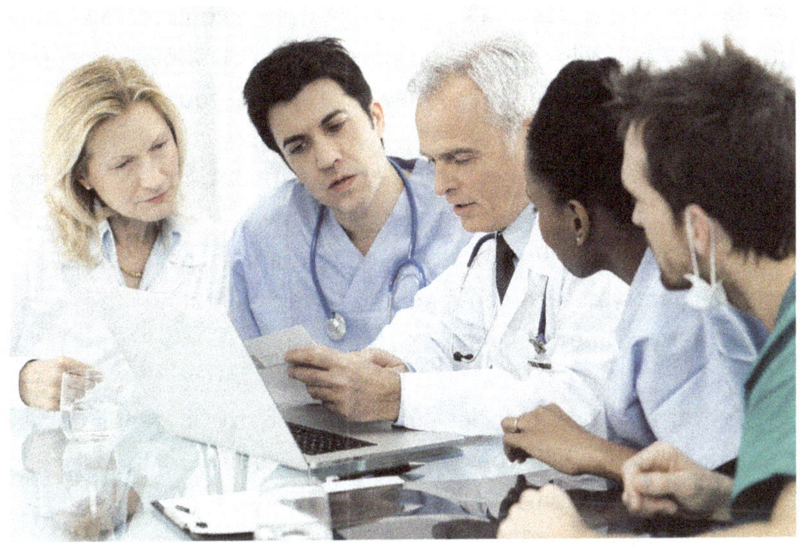

If you think you may be experiencing symptoms of an anxiety disorder, attack or related condition, please consult with your physician. He or she will be able to advise you if your symptoms match the clinical diagnosis of any of these mental health conditions.

If it is the case, you will need to consult with a professional that specializes in mental health conditions. These professionals are trained in therapy that deals with various behavioral patterns and will suggest medication if it is warranted.

Find one that you will be comfortable about discussing your condition with. You don't want to feel intimidated by their presence. You want to be relaxed and to be able to discuss what is going on with you. The mental health professional will work with you to devise a plan that will help you get over your struggles with these kinds of disorders and attacks.

If you are prescribed medication, you must take it as directed and don't stop unless you are advised by your physician. You and the mental health professional or your physician should discuss how the medication will work. If you have side effects, please consult them as soon as possible. They may have altered your dosage.

In regard to costs for medication and treatment, most insurance plans will cover that. However, don't assume and check with your insurance company first. If you lack insurance, check with your local or country government agency to seek mental health care at one of their facilities.

The governmental agencies usually stick to a sliding scale depending how much that you can pay. Or if you have public assistance, Medicaid may kick in to pay for these services.

Medication And Treatment

For the most part, medication is used for anxiety attacks, disorders and related conditions. The choices can depend on what the condition is and what the person wants. A physician must conduct a thorough evaluation to determine if they are indeed suffering from one of these mental health conditions.

If so, it must also be established as to what type of disorder they are dealing with. If there is a combination of things, they must also be identified so that the physician will know how to treat it.

If they have already received treatment from an existing or a past anxiety disorder condition, the physician needs to know that. They also need to know if medication was given and the dosage.

Or if they had other treatment, that needs to be disclosed as well. If there were any side effects, that should be included, along with any therapy that was provided and if it was beneficial for them.

There are some people that feel that the treatment they received did not work for them. Sometimes, it could be they may not have had enough time for the process to change or it was not done correctly. Some people may have to go through different medications or treatments to find what will work for them.

Medication is not the cure all for anxiety disorders, attacks and related conditions. However, medication can control these conditions while the person is receiving therapy. Medication can only be used if a physician prescribes it.

They are usually prescribed by psychiatrists that offer therapy of work with colleagues that provide some of the same services. For the most part, the medications that are used for anxiety disorders are:

•Antidepressants

•Anti-anxiety drugs

•Beta-blockers

Using any of these medications can help the person to live a normal life.

Antidepressants

Originally, antidepressants were used for treatment of depression. However, they also work for those that are suffering from anxiety disorders. They work to change the chemistry in the brain. Once the initial dose is taken, it takes at least 4 to 6 weeks before the symptoms will go away. The medication must be taken as directed in order for this to work.

• SSRIs – Selective Serotonin Reuptake Inhibitors – these antidepressants work to change the level of the communication of the brain cells. Some of the more common ones are Prozac, Zoloft and Lexapro.

They are used to treat any panic disorder that is mixed with social phobia, depression or OCD. Since these are newer, they don't have as many side effects. However, those that use them may experience being jittery or nauseated in the initial stages of taking them. This is only temporary.

• Tricycles – These antidepressants are older than SSRIs and are used for anxiety disorders other than OCD. They are administered with a low dosage and increase gradually.

Side effects include being dizzy, dry mouth, drowsy and weight gain. This can be eliminated by adjusting the dosage or using another medication of the same kind of antidepressant. Tofranil is used for GAD and panic disorder; Anafranil is used for OCD.

• MAOIs – Monoamine Oxidase Inhibitors – these are the oldest of the antidepressants available to use for these conditions. It is mostly used for anxiety disorders, attacks and related conditions.

Some of the more common ones are Nardil, Marplan and Parnate. When taking MAOIs, there are certain foods and drinks that you have to stay away from. That would include cheese and red wine.

In addition to that, you cannot take Advil, Motrin, Tylenol or any other pain, cold or allergy reliever medication. Plus, women will not be able to use certain types of birth control pills. Herbal supplements are also off limits. Mixing MAOIs with any of these can cause an adverse reaction.

• Anti-Anxiety Drugs – Drugs such as benzodiazepines are highly potent. They work to fight off anxiety and have very few side effects. Being drowsy is the only one that is noticeable. This drug is only prescribed for a brief period of time. Physicians are weary about providing them to past drug abusers.

Because people can get easily addicted to them, they look for additional doses so they can keep going. However, if the person has panic disorder, they can use these drugs up to a year.

For social phobia, Klonpin is used and Ativan is used for panic disorder. One of the most common antidepressants on the market is Xanax, which is used for GAD and panic disorder.

If a person stops taking benzodiazepines all of a sudden, they can experience withdrawals; the anxiety attacks can come back to haunt them. This is one reason why some physicians are leery about using this drug or use them sporadically.

Another anti-anxiety medication is Busiprone and it is used for GAD. There are some side effects that include nausea, headaches or dizziness. This is taken different than benzodiazepines. Busiprone has to be taken every day for at least two week before a person will feel the anti-anxiety effect from the drug.

• Beta-Blockers – Beta-blockers are used for treatment of heart conditions. They can also be used to keep away physical symptoms that determine anxiety disorders. Beta-blockers are used in situations such as if a person is giving a speech in front of other people, a bet-blocker can be used to keep those symptoms at bay.

How to Overcome Anxiety, Stress and Panic Naturally
If you are taking medication for an anxiety disorder, you should do the following:

• Have your physician to advise you on what medication would be effective for your condition.

• Have the physician consult you on how the drug works and what are the side effects from taking the drug.

• Inform your physician of other medications you may be taking. They may interfere with the dosage of the drug anxiety disorders.

The physician should advise you on the dosage and how you are directed to take it. They also need to advise you on how you should stop taking it when the time comes. With medication, some of them can actually trigger systems that can cause panic attacks. Physicians should always start out with a lower dose and then work their way up.

How to Overcome Anxiety, Stress and Panic Naturally Psychotherapy deals with interacting with a mental health professional, such as a psychologist, psychiatrist or someone who is trained in counseling of mental health issues and conditions. They can help to find out what triggers anxiety disorders and panic disorders. They also work to see what is the best path to take in order to combat the symptoms.

How to Overcome Anxiety, Stress and Panic Naturally Cognitive-Behavioral Therapy, or CBT, is very effective in the treatment of anxiety disorders. Thinking patterns are changed with the cognitive portion. The way people react to anxiety related issues is the behavioral portion.

People that have panic disorder can use cognitive-behavioral therapy to distinguish between heart attacks and panic attacks. CBT can also be used to help them overcome social phobia. It can help them to realize that everyone is not watching your every move, nor is everyone judging them.

There are techniques that they can learn to use for positive exposure. These techniques will also help them not to be so sensitive about anxiety triggers and symptoms.

 Therapy for those who suffer from is to get them to have contact with germs or dirt on their hands. They should wait around a while before they wash them. The therapist will help them deal with the anxiety that follows before they wash their hands. The more they do it, the more the anxiety goes away.

If a person suffers from social phobia, their therapy would be to spend time with others in social situations. They should resist trying to leave when they start to feel uncomfortable. They won't feel ashamed or feel that people are judging them.

If someone has PTSD, their therapy could be drumming up that event that caused them a lot of trauma and pain in their life. This can help to diminish the fear that they are feeling inside.

With cognitive-behavioral therapy, the therapists will provide ways of how you can implement deep breathing exercises and other exercises to get rid of anxiety. Exercises can help you to relax in tense and stressful situations.

Phobias have been treated with behavioral therapy that forces a person to expose themselves in a way that brings out their true fears and apprehensions. The face up to whatever it was that they feared.

It may be looking at photos or listening to voices on tape. It could also mean a face-to-face encounter with that person. The therapist will accompany them for support so that they can face their fears head on.

With CBT, this therapy must connect directly with the anxieties of the person and geared toward what they need. The only thing that will affect them is how uncomfortable they will feel because of the heightened anxiety. However, that is only temporary.

This type of therapy lasts for about three months or 12 weeks. It can be done as a one-on-one, or it can be with a group of people that are suffering from similar conditions. For social phobia, group therapy is better because a person will have to interact with other people. For certain anxiety disorders, medication may be required in order for the treatment to be effective.

Chapter 6- Alternative Way of Treating Anxiety

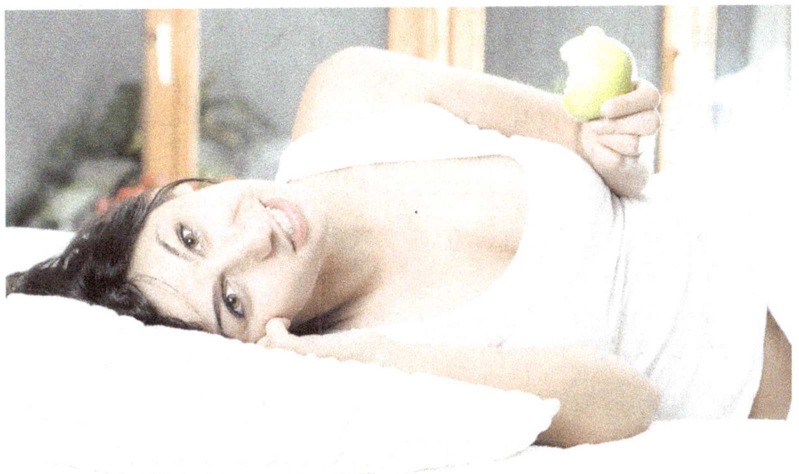

Other than taking medication and therapy, there are alternative treatments that can be used in order to combat these conditions in the anxiety and panic attack family.

One of the main keys to getting over anxiety and panic attacks is to relax. That's not as easy to do as some may think. Start out by focusing and making sure that you are breathing slowly and steadily.

When a person is having a panic attack, one of the first things that happens is they have trouble breathing. Sometimes they have to pant in order to catch their breath. The purpose here is to make your breaths even so that they will slow down your heart rate.

This will help the panic attack to eventually go away. A person is able to calm themselves by breathing slowly. They must continue to release air from their lungs. This helps to have deep breaths and make them feel calmer.

Lying down with your backside near a wall, bend the knees with the feet against the wall. Use one foot at a time and press into the wall. As you press it in, breathe in. As you release it from the wall, breathe out. Change up your feet when you are doing this. Take about 15 minutes until the feeling of panic has lifted from you.

Try not to think about the past. A lot of times, panic attacks happen from something that has to do with your past that you were upset about. Look at different shapes and colors. If you like pets, get a small dog or cat and love on it.

If you are into fragrances, you can use aromatherapy to relieve yourself of anxiety and panic attacks. One aroma that has a calming effect is lavender. There are many places where you can purchase essential oils.

When you feel an anxiety or panic attack coming on, sniff the oil and it will work to calm you down. You can also use it as massage oil, along with olive or grape seed oil. There are other aromatherapy oils you can use. You have to smell them to see which one you prefer.

How To Make Your Treatment More Effective

There are independent support groups that you can join. You will be able to share your knowledge and experience with those who are dealing with similar problems. There are also chat rooms online.

However, this has to be done with caution. Not everything someone says about anxiety and panic attacks are the gospel. You can also seek the counsel of your pastor of minister of the cloth. However, you need to make sure that you seek counseling from a trained mental health professional.

There are also meditation and techniques that deal with managing stress. This can help those with these disorders so that you can stay calm and focused. This can also help with your therapy. As you are finding ways to find peace within yourself, there are some things that you should avoid consuming.

They would include beverages that have caffeine, illegal drugs and some cold and sinus medications from over the counter. They can actually provoke the symptoms of anxiety and panic disorders.

Your family is crucial to have in your life in order for you to make a full recovery. They should be supportive and help you in every way they can. However, there may be some family members that may want to deride and ridicule you.

They may tend to think that is trivial and has no merit. You may have speak with them and get them to understand that this is a serious condition. If they still refuse, then move on and find some friends that will have your back and provide you with the support that you need.

Panic Attacks That Are Left Untreated

Panic attacks can continue for a long time, sometimes for years to come. This longevity can be complicated by having consistent attacks. Symptoms include having certain phobias (fears) or leaving outside the home, not wanting to be around other people, feeling suicidal, financial issues and substance abuse. As a result, the person could end up suffering from heart disease.

If the panic attacks are not treated, the anxiety can increase and get worse. Their daily routine may be affected by attacks that are not going away. This must be dealt with head on; otherwise, the person cannot be a productive citizen of society.

How to Prevent Panic Attacks

There are ways that you can decrease the chance of an onset of a panic attack. You can learn how to deal with them better. You must recognize the symptoms. When the initial ones begin, they may be others that come along. Just remember to take slow and deep breaths.

Keep decreasing you anxiety level through things such as exercise and meditation. Don't be in a rush and take your time with this. Doing it quickly can defeat the purpose. Therapy is a time consuming process and improvement will be gradual.

Don't be hard on yourself. Take it easy. Don't beat yourself over the head criticizing yourself because of your condition. Make sure that you avoid things such as cigarettes, teas that have caffeine, and carbonated drinks. That may be difficult, but at least start weaning your way off slowly.

Work on not thinking about things that may have been traumatic for you in the past. These traumatic events can shape how you will react to things in the future. You cannot allow the past to hinder you if you are looking to move forward.

Make sure to keep a loving and understanding support system around you so that you will be able to move forward every day. Whether it's family members or a friend, they need to be genuinely interested in help you get better and relieve those fears that you have pent up inside.

How To Lend Your Support

If you are helping someone who has one of these conditions, it is very important that you are there for the long haul. It may take longer than a few weeks or months for that person to totally overcome this.

You should not be judgmental or condescending in any way to the person who is suffering. This is a serious matter and you should treat it as such. The worst thing you could do regarding anxiety and panic attacks is to be dismissive and think that they can quickly get over it. You cannot be the savior for them and solve their problem.

People who suffer these kinds of attacks are not thinking about anything except how scared they are that something bad is going to happen. The situation cannot be solved by shaking them and making them come out of it, or waving a magic wand over them and saying "abracadabra".

Don't underestimate their actions by thinking that they are pretending to be acting. This is serious and their actions should not be underestimated. The best thing you can do is to do everything in your power that you can to be there as that support system.

They could feel at any moment that they were in grave danger. They feel as though they could not pull themselves out of whatever trouble they perceived. This Is when the accelerated heartbeat, shortness of breath and other symptoms come in to play.

If you ignore them, you are doing more to hurt them than to help. They depend on your support and if you decide to bail out on their weakest moment, they will feel more worthless.

This could make them start feeling depressed and not want to do much of anything for their situation. If they know that you are with them to help them stick it out, then they will feel better about themselves.

You must allow them to go through the attack. If you try to intervene, you could make the situation worse. Let it happen and they will eventually come out of it. However, if for some reason they don't stop, call a paramedic to assist.

One thing that you don't want to do is to give them medication, especially if it's not prescribed by their physician. That will definitely cause them harm. So make sure that you are not doing anything to jeopardize their well being.

There is hope for those who have been suffering for a long time with anxiety disorders, attacks, and panic attacks. You have to be willing to make the move to make changes in your life. There are other people out there that are suffering just like you.

However, your situation doesn't have to stay this way forever. There is help out there in the form of medication, and therapy. You just have to want it for yourself. The sooner you get the help, the better you will get. Once you do that, you will stop allowing these conditions to control your life.

CHAPTER 7- DON'T LET ANXIETY ATTACKS DICTATE YOU

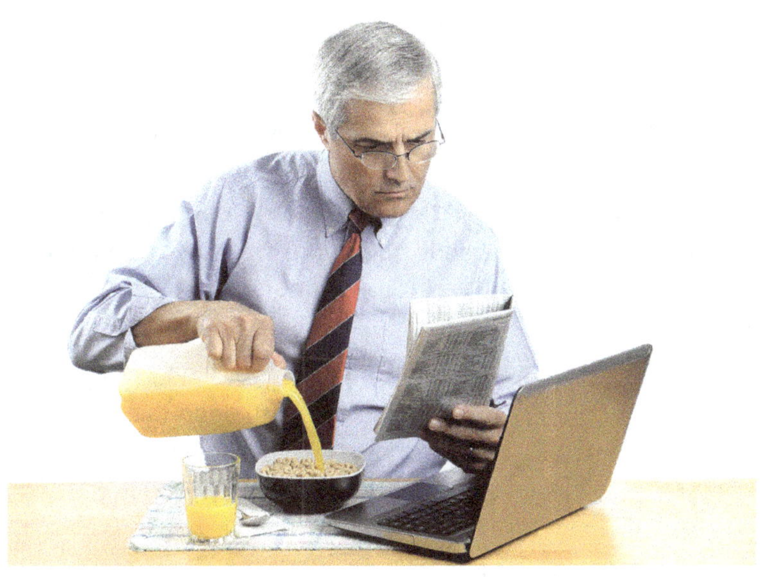

Every important journey begins with the first few steps, and often these first few steps are the most difficult Overcoming Social Anxiety disorder is no different. Even when we realize we truly need a change, that we need to do those things that others before us have done to become better, beginning the pathway to change can be challenging.

There are a few things we can keep in mind and tips to follow that can help. I can't guarantee that they will make the first few steps easy - making that type of promise to a person with Social Anxiety disorder would be insincere, What I do know is that despite initial discomfort they will make the first big hurdle of breaking inertia possible to get over. They've worked again and again for people with even the worst phobias. They'll most likely work for you too!

Clearly Establish Change is Necessary

The first thing that you need to come to terms with yourself more than anyone else is just how necessary change is. If you have a big enough "Why" getting through the "How" end of things is fueled by real desire.

This motivating force should never be underestimated. Sit down with a pen and paper and write down the areas that your Social Anxiety disorder is having a negative influence on. Turn the page and write your dreams that you can more easily achieve without Social Anxiety disorder handcuffing your ability to communicate establish relationships and take action.

When this is complete read over both lists for as long as it takes for these truths to REALLY sink in. When you are done this should give both your conscious and subconscious mind the foundation it needs to support your effort to cure your Social Anxiety.

Find a Plan and Stick with It

One of the real obstacles to making lasting positive change in life (which is exactly the area where curing Social Anxiety disorder falls into) is lack of commitment.

You can find many different ideas on how to ease social phobias including those presented here in our Guide. Almost all will work to varying degrees if you work their method and stick with it until you see positive results. What doesn't work is trying something for a few days and allowing impatience to seize control and immediately jumping to a different program.

Choose a plan to fight your Social Anxiety disorder, stick to it and give it a chance to work. If you need a bit of extra motivation think of the story of the man who was mining for gold and stopped only a few inches away from what would have been his big discovery only to return to a life of poverty. Self help can often be the same way. Don't change plans like you change socks - give the work a chance to work!

Start Sooner Rather than Later

It's pretty likely you have suffered from Social Anxiety disorder for way too long. The final pieces of advice I have on beginning the pathway to change are to not over think things and begin today. Once you are on the path and begin gaining momentum you are that much closer to freedom! Letting "doing it" beat out "thinking about it".

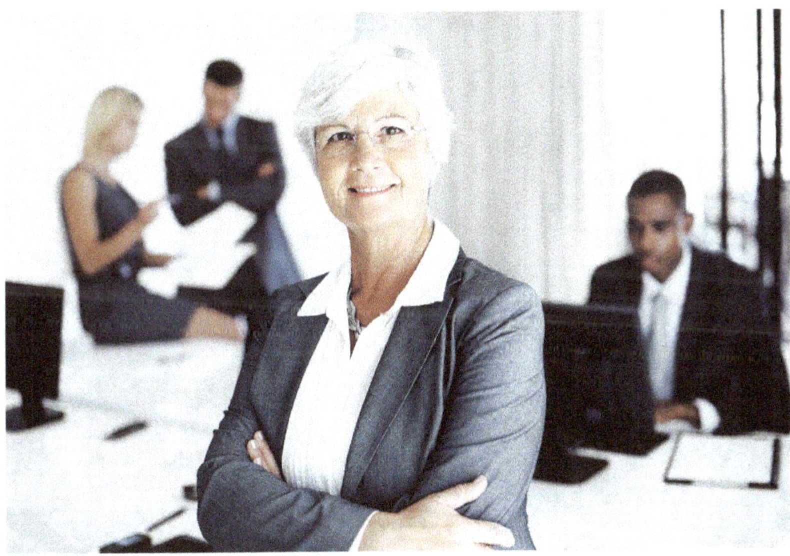

About the Author

Steven Edwards had a rough teenage life. He had anxiety attacks every time that he is in a crowd or during school activities that requires an audience. For some reason he had this feeling that he can't be able to explain. Thus, starts the panicking, shortness of breath, nausea and other related discomforts.

With the help of their guidance counselor and a family friend, Edwards was able to manage his condition and become a very successful entertainer and an author of several books.

He lives in Denver, Colorado with his wife and two lovely daughters.

www.ingramcontent.com/pod-product-compliance
Lightning Source LLC
Chambersburg PA
CBHW070052260726

48658CB00002B/861

ECONOMICS MADE SIMPLE

A PERFECT GUIDE FOR ECONOMICS

VIPUL BAIBHAV

Copyright © Vipul Baibhav
All Rights Reserved.

ISBN 978-1-63850-791-8

This book has been published with all efforts taken to make the material error-free after the consent of the author. However, the author and the publisher do not assume and hereby disclaim any liability to any party for any loss, damage, or disruption caused by errors or omissions, whether such errors or omissions result from negligence, accident, or any other cause.

While every effort has been made to avoid any mistake or omission, this publication is being sold on the condition and understanding that neither the author nor the publishers or printers would be liable in any manner to any person by reason of any mistake or omission in this publication or for any action taken or omitted to be taken or advice rendered or accepted on the basis of this work. For any defect in printing or binding the publishers will be liable only to replace the defective copy by another copy of this work then available.